THE COMPLETE #2020 INTERMITTENT FASTING BOOK

Lose Weight with Quick and Healthy Recipes
For Every Day incl. 16:8 and 5:2 Diet Plan

MATTHEW MORGAN

Copyright © [2019] [Matthew Morgan]

All rights reserved

All rights for this book here presented belong exclusively to the author. Usage or reproduction of the text is forbidden and requires a clear consent of the author in case of expectations.

ISBN- 9798613039388

TABLE OF CONTENTS

Introduction 7

    Pros of intermittent fasting 8

    How does fasting work? 10

    The different fasting methods 12

    How does the 16:8 method work 15

    Where do I have to pay attention? 20

Example of 16/8 menu for 7 days 26

Experience 28

Recommended food by dieticians for 5/2 diet 33

    Examples of menu for 2 days 37

Personal experience 38

Goal Setting 43

    Set yourself on healthy food 46

    Aspects to be taken into consideration while dieting 48

30 healthy recipes on intermittent fasting + 30 interesting facts … 51

1 day … 51

- Chicken with broccoli … 52
- Salad with bacon and pasta … 54
- Tuna Avocado Salad … 56
- Mongolian Tofu … 58
- Avocado salad with beans and eggs … 60
- Baked salmon with vegetables … 62
- Cheese soup … 64
- Protein spinach pancakes … 66
- Pumpkin cream soup … 67
- Eggs' muffins with black beans … 69
- Meatballs with spinach … 71
- Chicken salad with apples and cranberry … 73
- Turkey muffins with broccoli … 75
- Prawns with rice in tomato sauce … 77
- Banana pudding … 79
- Spaghetti with vegetables … 81
- Ratatouille … 83
- Carrot sugar free cake … 85
- Tomato puree soup … 87

Lentil with vegetables 89
Baked chicken with spinach 91
Cheese Casserole with pumpkin 93
Lean beans cutlets 95
Stuffed peppers 97
Broccoli casserole 99
Chicken sandwich 101
Vegetarian rolls 103
Chocolate chip cookies 105
Granola bars 107
Zucchini casserole 109

Disclaimer 110

INTRODUCTION

Intermittent fasting -is a nutrition system, a way to organize your menu so that to make the most use of it. A lot of Hollywood stars prefer this diet and point out good results such as actors Hugh Jackman, Benedict Cumberbatch and Justin Theroux, Beyoncé singer and model Miranda Kerr are in an excellent shape and don't hide that use this fat loss method.

This is an effective method of weight loss, that lies in refusing from food now and again. Such kind of nutrition induces body to burn extra fat stocks. The main advantage of intermittent fasting is that you don't have to refrain from food at all, it is well enough to skip breakfast, lunch or dinner. Emotionally it is much easier than a complete fasting or for instance fast days on juices. In fact, there are no limits in products. That means you can afford yourself some cheat meals like desserts, bread, baking goods, fried food etc.

The concept of intermittent fasting that optimizes insulin secretion and it makes organism less sensitive to carbohydrates of high Glycemic Index, decreases hunger. At the moment of fasting your organism starts to burn fat reserve without distracting itself on food processing. Furthermore, empty stomach can «chill out», it increases immune system and improves hormonal. Some nutritionists are sure that such kind of diet diminishes inflammatory processes in body, regulates sugar level in blood and boosts your mental activity. In conjunction with intermittent fasting and power workout you may gain muscle mass on account burning fat the body will be more strong and fit.

Pros of intermittent fasting

First of all it is a smart decision to lose weight without following strict diet and cutting down on calories to zero.

✓ **Well-structured schedule**
Intermittent fasting allows to make day steady and spend less time on cooking and eating.

✓ **Positive effect on heath condition.**
Limiting calories is a way of continuing life. Intermittent fasting activates lots of mechanisms that prolong life.

✓ **Intermittent fasting can decrease the risk of developing diseases.**
A lot of investigations have shown that fasting not only reduces risk Cancer, Alzheimer's disease, but also cardiovascular disease

✓ **Intermittent fasting is more simple and effective than diet.**

The reason why most diets don't show a desirable result not because we consume wrong food but we don't follow diet during long-term period. This kind of diet creates a habit and ensures a great outcome.

✓ **Prevents senility process and promotes growing new nerve cells.**

As every diet fasting has also contraindications, so before doing experiments with your body you should consult with a doctor. Intermittent fasting is forbidden for people who suffer from

- Gastritis
- Diabetes
- Low pressure
- Gallbladder problems
- Adrenals problems

And also fasting is not recommended for

- Underweight people
- Breastfeeding mothers
- Pregnant woman

How does fasting work?

During 8-10 hour period you afford yourself 3 meals, and then you eat nothing during 14-16 hours. The simplest way of following intermittent fasting system is that you can skip meals on your discretion. For example from 8am-16pm you can eat 2-3 meals from healthy ration of nutrition and after 16pm-8am you can dine and count down 8-10 hours since this moment. As soon as they passed you can come back to normal eating.

At the time of fasting you can drink water, tea, coffee. It is forbidden to consume drinks that contain calories coffee with sugar, milk and cream, smoothie juices sparkling water or any alcohol.

Everything is quite clear. Fasting works perfectly and aids to slim down quickly thanks to quick restart of digestion system, gives time to relax and repair.

System 16/8 works as an intermittent fasting so it can be practiced 1-2 times per week.

Firstly, this system is good for sustaining a good physical shape. When an organism switches over hungry regime it launches a process of the splitting of fat instead of glucose -this natural mechanism allowed our ancestors to live through food shortage and modern human to get rid of overeating outcomes.

Secondly, autophagy process is reinforced-disposing from dead cells and their particles in conjunction with strengthened production of growth hormone. Particularly it occurs at the time of sleeping which also counts as one of the fasting effects and gives a potent incentive to cells regeneration.

Thirdly, intermittent fasting has a positive impact on sugar level in your blood. Particularly it is topical for people who have it increased, including people sick in 2d type diabetes. (It is forbidden to fast having 1 type diabetes.)Insulin level is normalized and cells' sensitivity is restored to it and to hormone leptin which is responsible for appetite control, satiety and hunger signals. Resistance (decreasing of these 2 hormones) is a sign of metabolism syndrome- metabolism disorder that leads to different health problems and also promotes to a rapid visceral fat gain. As opposed to subcutaneous fat deposits it accumulates on internal organs near stomach and boosts the risk of cardiovascular and endocrine diseases. It is quite complicated to get rid of it with the help of a usual diet so intermittent fasting regularly based will kill it quite successfully.

In addition, people who suffer from digestion problems due to a lazy bowel peristalsis or sick microbiome in, starving can help and dramatically improve situation. For the time of starving all inflammatory processes are disappeared (it regards not only digestion system) and fermentation process as well. Some professors approve that just this time is the best for consuming probiotics to achieve maximal effect in minimal terms.

The different fasting methods

Over the last few years intermittent fasting has taken the world by storm and become extremely trendy. It is proved that it promotes losing weight, enhances metabolism health. Taking into consideration popularity, it is no wonder that several different methods or types of intermittent fasting have been created recently. Every method can be effective but which of them works out the best, depends on a person.

Here are 6 most famous and important ways of fasting

1. **16/8 Method**- this kind of intermittent fasting suggests eating during 8-10 hours and after you consume no food during 14-16 hours. During eating window you are allowed to eat 2-3 or more meals. Such system is very simple and in fact you eat nothing after dinner and skip breakfast. If you can't do without breakfast it will be difficult for you to get used to such kind of diet. This is one of the most natural methods of intermittent fasting and doesn't require big efforts. This method we will consider more in details a bit later.

2. **5/2 Method**- this method offers 5 days of usual nutrition and restrictions to 500-600 calories for 2 days in a week. This Method of intermittent fasting was established by British journalist Michael Mosley. Usually people divide their fast days into a week. For example they go fasting on Monday and Thursday and in other days eat normally. It is recommended to have at least 1 non-fasting

day between fasting days. This diet decreases insulin level and diminishes weight.

3. **Alternate day fasting**-it is basically kind of intermittent fasting, this method requires to alternate meals and fasting hours. According to this program you can fast several hours or the whole day and even longer. ADF is considered to be one of the most extreme fasting periods. It was defined as a strict 36-day period without consuming calories in a magazine «Cell Metabolism» In fact it means that you don't eat for 36 hours and then eat everything you want during the rest 12 hours.

4. **A weekly 24-hour fast**-complete fasting during 1-2 days per week is well-known as «eat-stop-eat» involves not only food during 24 hour simultaneously. A lot of people fast from breakfast till breakfast or from lunch till lunch. People following this regime can drink water or other calorie-free beverages.24-hour fasting can be quite complicated for newbies; they can experience, irritability headache or fatigue. Some researchers approve that these effects become less extreme in the long run, when organism gets accustomed to this new scheme/pattern of nutrition. For the first time it may be easier to give a try to 12-16 hour fasting before going to 24 hour fasting.

5. **Meal omitting**-this flexible approach to IF can be useful for newbies. It provides meal skipping now and again. Probably it will be the most suitable for people who keep an eye and react on the

starvation signals of their organism. Some people find this method easier and more natural than other methods.

6. **The Warrior Diet**-this nutrition system was offered by artist and former riot policeman Ori Hofmekler. This diet suggests eating a few raw vegetables and fruits during the day and in the evening – a substantial meal. In fact you fast the whole day (20 hours) and before going to bed you have an opportunity to have a big meal. The Warrior diet has become one of the first and popular diets which applied method of intermittent fasting. The selection of products reminds «paleo diet»-consuming of whole unprocessed products.

16/8 Method- this method involves daily fasting during 14-16 hours and restricting «eating-window» up to 8-10 hours. This method is well-known as protocol Leangains and was established by fitness expert Martin Berkhan.

How does the 16:8 method work

Cyclical way of nutrition is quite liberal: a person can ascertain his time restrictions depending on personal biorhythms and every day circumstances by himself. If you are an early bird -it will be easier for you to eat for example from 8 am-4p.m. or from 9am.-5pm. The suitable time for night owls- is from 12am-8pm.

You can eat allowed products, and for boosting your activity and launching metabolism processes it is recommended to include in your nutrition schedule –workout. Every morning it is necessary to make time for active physical exercises in order to improve result.

Despite that this diet allows to eat everything you long for, there is a row of products recommended to include in the ration of your nutrition 8/16 with a view to receiving not only gone calories but to boost up your health too. We can divide them in 2 categories:

Fat-burning:

- Lean, non-fat meat(chicken, turkey, rabbit, eggs)
- Nuts(almond and walnuts),raw pumpkin seeds
- Beans, pea, chickpea
- Dairy products with low-fat content(plain yogurt)

Health-improving/recreational:

- Blue and red berries: cherry, currant ,blackberry
- Fiber and antioxidant sources: citruses, apples.
- Green vegetables and rabbit food, all kinds of cabbage, cucumbers, spinach etc.
- Carotenoids, lycopene-containing vegetables: tomatoes, carrot, bell pepper.

It is recommended to include at least 1-2 products from both groups. The amount of consumed carbohydrates must be minimized or excluded at all. But if you can't do without them, mix pasta with non-fat cheese and vegetables, cornflakes with milk and fruits, and add bread to lean meat and salad. You should also cut down on alcohol and drink a plenty of water.

How to prepare yourself to fasting

1. Make a plan of nutrition per week.

2. Don't try to restrict yourself in everything-distribute calories properly.

3. The most important value of meals wholly, a person must intake food filled with useful and nutritious properties. However you don't have to refrain from fast and junk food entirely, you should practice your moderation, healthy habits and skills to focus on more healthy choices to make most of it.

16/8 diet Advantages
- Sound sleep
- Metabolism improvement
- Stabilization of food habits
- Proper nutrition
- Simple existing version for newbies
- Conscious food consumption
- Strict restriction absence
- Quick result

16/8 diet disadvantages
- Not everybody bears such food restrictions
- For the first time people can experience frequent hunger sense
- Fatigue
- Lack of mood

- The complexity of implementing for example for office workers

Main rules

- ✓ Firstly, before following this diet you should adjust your schedule and sleep pattern. You won't see results without that. So think in advance what time you are being active and energetic.
- ✓ Choose the best time for fasting and nutrition. Take into account your schedule. Try to think when do you always eat. Attempt to make your schedule so that your favorite time for eating hasn't disappeared. Of course it is not recommended to eat before sleep. It is better to eat for 2-3 hours before going to bed.
- ✓ Always give your organism to wake up after sleep, drink a cup of water on empty stomach, intake vitamins and take up some exercises. After 2-3 hours you can eat.
- ✓ Countdown commences since your breakfast. For instance, if you ate at 10am so you need to acquire your personal calories till 6pm. Your fasting starts after 6pm. Before sleep you may drink plain yogurt or milk if you are not hungry then don't do that. It is desirable to fall asleep before 10-11pm therefore you won't be hungry and will stick to proper sleep pattern.
- ✓ Actually, it is quite complicated to eat all calories during 8 hours because most of people just can't make it according to different life rhythms. However, the more active you are the better. Thanks to all your activity during the day calories are burnt faster. You shouldn't miss meals or rearrange them for a couple hours. Take food along

with you, so-called «packed snacks», take into account that if you don't eat and miss one of meals you won't be able to eat during the day. This threatens of having a breakdown in best case, nausea, throwing up and other serious spillover effects.

Time frames and potential achievements

As you have already seen above there exist different kinds of intermittent fasting. Indeed there is rougher for example 18/6 and more relaxed that people live and stick to even not being aware of it.

Talking about time frames –everybody makes up his mind by himself if this diet will be a trial period or current lifestyle. Anyway you have to stop a diet if you feel bad.

Potential achievements

- For week-2-3kg
- For 14days-5-6 days
- For month 8-10kg
- For 2 months-10 kg

Intermittent fasting gives following results:

- Decreasing insulin level which helps organism to use accumulated fat
- Reducing sugar-level in blood and arterial pressure

- Body activates process which is called «autophagy» that means that organism digests or recycles old or damaged cells.

In a research which was published in a magazine «Nutrition and healthy senility», it was firstly studied influence of limited meal on people with obesity or excess weight. Researchers worked with 23 patients suffering from obesity. Each of them reached 45 age. The participants were allowed to eat any food in any amount between 10am-6pm. During the rest hours they could drink only water or other low calorized drinks. The investigation had been lasting for 12 weeks and received name diet 16/8 because contestants ate only 8 hours and during 16 hours were fasting. It was discovered that those participants who stuck to diet, gradually lost weight and improved blood pressure. People lost 3% of their total weight. Results have shown that without counting calories and limiting harmful products it is possible to achieve wanted effect.

Where do I have to pay attention?

However 16/8 fasting doesn't require to avoid and eat definite products; it is advisable to concentrate on proper nutrition and avoid consuming harmful and unhealthy food. Consumption of excess fast and junk food can cause increasing weight and promote illnesses.

- **Well-balanced diet** focused on firstly fruits, vegetables, whole grains that contain a lot of fiber so it will help a person to feel herself

- satisfied and full-fledged. Healthy fats and proteins will make you full for a long time.

- Before start you should **set your objectives** .It is important to ask yourself what are your personal goals regarding diet. If you strive to promote healthy senility or just reach more healthy weight. Different aims succumb in different plans so awareness of what are you going to receive from this diet will help you do choose the best choice.

- **Also you must be ready for some failures** because there is no 1 plan that works out for all people. You should choose the most suitable variant for u. Based on narrations of your friends or relatives you cannot be sure that just this diet will be good and effective for you. Even when make all your investigations you can detect that the plan you stick to doesn't work out for you. Being a lot of time without food may cause irritability and may not work with your schedule. It is significant to be aware of how your daily routine and intermittent fasting work altogether and according to it adjust

- As a matter of fact you should **work your way up**. Probably you have heard about considerable benefits that come with 16 hour fasting but maybe you have no desire to deepen in to it right away. It has been mentioned in a report that the best way to nail your plan is to ease it and not to dive your head in an aggressive plan entirely. It will give your organism enough time to get used to new schedule which may differ from your former food habits.

Kick off from less frequent fasting plan with an intention to draw up more intensive program if you intend to reach a success with IF in the long run.

- **Pay attention on your body.** One of the most important parts of solving a problem connected with health and healthy loss weight is a persuasion that you adjust yourself on feelings that you perceive in new procedures. For some people intermittent fasting cannot the best choice. There are some traps you may get in which may cause health problems.

- Also you should pay attention on **stress level** in your life because it may remove all good results. Any change of routine may lead to a stress and start of IF is undoubtedly a change in a schedule. According to some researching, fasting may trigger stress hormone « cortisol ».The principle of stress eating may have some truth and disrupt your fasting plan.

- **Try to keep a diary.** Keeping a record of what you eat may help you better keep track of how different meals cause various feelings and it was shown that it is a potential way for increasing advantages for losing weight after fasting. But there is no need in taking notes of all food you consume, it may be also useful to monitor your spirit and other factors because it may help you to observe your progress you reach and make you adjust on innate indicators of your body. This is an excellent way to assure yourself that you won't become a victim of widespread intermittent fasting mistakes just making yourself more responsible.

- If talking about intermittent fasting **woman have sundry needs.** Intermittent fasting may influence on man's and woman's hormones but woman's hormones are more sensitive to fasting signals that may lead to boosting level of hunger. It's no wonder that it complicates following a plan so it is critical to be aware of these outcomes. Because of this reason some doctors recommend woman to follow a plan that predicts a gradual increasing of fasting not abrupt start of a plan.
- Also it is necessary to give special attention to **physical exercises.** If you are going to work out you should think beforehand what to eat depending on the training intensity. For example you can build up your glycogen stores with complex carbohydrates for the dinner to have an energy for training.
- It is not recommended to train on empty stomach because sudden demand on a bloodstream from muscles will steal vital blood flow which is necessary for digestion system in order to metabolize and absorb nutrient supply. The most important is to plan in advance to make your nutrition to fit the demands required by intensity of your workout

Main rules

- **8-hour window choice**-(restrict consuming food in given period of time, set it on your own according to your schedule, for example 9am-5pm)

- **Smaller meals**-(to keep your hunger under the control and to stabilize sugar blood level it is recommended to consume food in small portions equally distributed during your eating window.
- **Allowed products**-(to achieve better results you should draw up your ration exclusively from whole nutritious products)
- **Liquid consuming**-(water, sugar free tea, coffee, juices, it will help to stay hydrated during the day)
- **8-hour sleep is compulsory**
- **Fresh air**-(there is a better way to improve training hours jogging in a park instead of gym)

Tips

- People may find/bear/endure process of fasting more easily just following next recommendations
- Stay hydrated during the day. Drink herbal cinnamon tea during the fasting because it may take the edge of appetite and consume a plenty of water regularly.
- Avoid food obsession. Plan a bunch of things to do, to avoid thoughts about food.
- Time off and relax. Avoid tensed occupations during fasting days, although light exercises such as yoga can be extremely useful.
- Watch less TV for reducing the exposure food images that may stimulate feeling/sense of hunger

- Take up exercising before «window meal because physical power work out may trigger appetite
- If chosen plan allows a bit calories during fasting days choose products that contain fat substances rich in proteins, fiber and healthy fats ,like beans, lentil, eggs, fish, nuts, avocado.
- Boosting taste without calories. You can generously season meals with garlic powder, herbs, spices or vinegar. These products have extremely less caloric value and filled with flavor that may help to take the edge of your appetite.
- Practice smart eating during meal
- Try to meditate during fasting to remove hunger pangs

Feedback of a girl who experienced this diet

«Having analyzed my own feelings I can say that it is an excellent system for people who love relatively big portions by dint to feel comfort and lightness. Also swollen is gone and body becomes more mobile. There is no hunger sense because meals were quite caloric and there is no constant desire to chew something»

Example of 16/8 menu for 7 days

All recipes you may find in our bonus chapter «4 Weeks Weight Loss Meal Plan»

Day 1

8:00 am: 1 cup of water

8.30 am: Skip breakfast

12.00 am: Chicken with broccoli

3:00pm: Nuts

7:00pm: Salad with bacon and pasta

8:00pm: Begin fasting

Day 2

8:00 am: Lemon water

8.30 am: Skip breakfast

12.00 am: Avocado Tuna salad

3:00pm: Apple

7:00pm: Mongolian Tofu

8:00pm: Begin fasting

Day 3

8:00 am: black coffee

8.30 am: Skip breakfast

12.00 am: Avocado salad with beans and eggs

3:00pm: Pear

7:00pm: Baked salmon with vegetables

8:00pm: Begin fasting

Day 4

8:00 am: Lemon water

8.30 am: Skip breakfast

12.00 am: Cheese soup

3:00pm: pumpkin seeds

7:00pm: Protein spinach pancakes

8:00pm: Begin fasting

Day 5

8:00 am: green tea

8.30 am: Skip breakfast

12.00 am: Pumpkin cream soup

3:00pm: Blueberries

7:00pm: eggs muffins with beans

8:00pm: Begin fasting

Day 6

8:00 am: Water

8.30 am: Skip breakfast

12.00 am: Meatballs with spinach

3:00pm: Greek yogurt

7:00pm: Chicken salad with apples and cranberry
8:00pm: Begin fasting

Day 7
8:00 am: Warm honey lemon water
8.30 am: Skip breakfast
12.00 am: Turkey muffins with broccoli
3:00pm: Granola bar
7:00pm: Prawns with rice in tomato sauce
8:00pm: Begin fasting

Experience

Intermittent fasting 16/8 has helped doctor to lose 57 kg for 18 months.

When most of diets have a plenty of/a number of rules and difficulties, intermittent fasting makes weight loss simple matter. It's no wonder that such way of weight control gain more fans in the whole world. Even doctors take advantage of this diet.

Kevin Gendreau is a doctor who used this method of fasting and managed to lose 57kg for 18 months. Before a person starts acting a turning point in his life may happen. This crucial moment came for doctor when his sister passed away because of cancer.

Observing how disease gradually took her life away, doctor began to think of his own life. At that moment his weight was 136kg with 160cm height.

«My poor sister had no choice. I decided to be healthy»

Kevin started to put on weight being a student. He gained additional 23kg because of a stress. When his father deceased, food became a comfort source for him. Young doctor kept on getting fat during several years.

«Gradually you fall in despair and lose your faith in capability to control your emotions and hunger. I had no idea how strong my moderation. However, observing how my sister was fighting with cancer, I understood that just wrong lifestyle became the reason of my own health problems like high pressure and increased level of cholesterol, diabetes»

As soon as he realized it, something just clicked in his head and Kevin managed to concentrate on slimming down.

In august 2016, he cut out all simple carbohydrates and started consuming 1700 calories per day. First 18 kg just melted immediately. Then doctor looked through his ration of nutrition more thoroughly, focusing on following

- ✓ Vegetables
- ✓ Beans
- ✓ Sugar free black coffee
- ✓ Non-fat Greek yogurt

- ✓ Fruits
- ✓ Nuts

Ration change has helped man to lose more weight. But as soon as scales showed 100g, his progress stopped. Only after sister's death in June 2017 he kept on dieting and training. He used well-known 16/8 fasting.

«I felt much better, but when my sister's condition worsened, it motivated me not to stop on achieved.

He ate everything he wanted from 12 am-8p.m and then took a break.

It helped him to get rid of the rest of 27kg.

«90%of my weight loss is a diet»

In general his slimming took 18m months.

«I am struck it really works out. Intermittent fasting is extremely healthy and efficient diet that I loved»

What's now? Last couple of months Kevin started intensively working out. He hopes that physical exercises will help to firm up saggy skin. Kevin goes on slimming and is going to reach healthy body mass index in the short run. He doesn't take pills anymore and feels himself completely healthy.

Method 5/2-

Method 5/2- involves restricting of consumed calories for 25 percent energy needs, 2 days per week and the rest of the week normal eating. That means the less you consume calories the more you slim down. It allows eating everything you want 5 days in a week and the rest 2 days men have to restrict their ration to 600 calories and woman to 500 calories.

2 main conditions:
- ✓ fast days don't have to be adjoining
- ✓ Break between meals must be at least 12 hours.

In a month people can lose their weight to 3 kg and in half a year-nearly 10kg. In addition part-time food refusal includes gen-recovery due to which organism starts to get rid of old and damaged cells. The author of this nutrition system is Kerry Torens, specialist BBC in terms of nutritious branch assures that this diet is useful not only for people who suffer from excess weight but also for those who want to keep good health condition and upgrade well-being.

The system of nutrition is effective because of simple physiological component. The fat in a human body starts to burn when the more energy is spent than is consumed. Nevertheless medium value of spent energy is counted for 3 days at least not for 24 hour.

Perfect choice - breakfast at 7 o'clock and dinner at 7 o'clock. It is counted that just this term in essential for organism to switch from fat accumulating regime to fat burning regime. The concept of nutrition shows that there is no need in strict limiting but also it doesn't mean that you have to eat only junk and fast food. Include in your ration more green vegetables, protein and healthy fats.

How does 5/2 method work?

Firstly Michael Moskley successfully tested this diet on himself and only then exposed it in his publishment. The results didn't make to wait. During 6 weeks of this system 5 days normal eating (2000 calories per day) and 2 days (no more than 500-600 calories) he managed to get rid of 6 kg)

Don't forget about the main rule of this diet - fast days don't have to be adjoining(!)So for example, you can choose Tuesday and Saturday or any other days, personally suitable for everyone. As a result decreasing ration of nutrition 2 times per week, the body gets not big but still stress, activating fat burning process of accumulated fat. Just short-term jolts which are more effective than long-term tantalizing diets, as at the time of permanent restrictions the human body starts getting accustomed to new conditions and as a result weight loss comes to an end.

Modifications

It's not easy to switch from normal eating every day to 500-600 calories every day per 2 days. Instead of doing such jolt you may to try consuming calories more slowly. For example during 1 week cut down on calories from 2000 calories to 1500.Next week try to eat 1000 calories. Keep on decreasing by smaller steps until you eat recommended 500-600 calories in fasting days.

Main rules

- You can eat bread, fruits, meat, vegetables and fish
- It is forbidden to exceed 500 calories during fast days.
- It's not recommended to eat chocolate, sparkling water, alcohol; it can be replaced with soups, porridges, cereals. If it is hard for u to refuse from such treatment you can choose healthy desserts
- It is better to steam food, boil, bake or stew.
- You have to eat more fiber, useful sugar free products

Fat loss period must go gradually without weight hikes. You don't have to follow this nutrition system for the rest of your life. It is not a style- it is express-method.

Recommended food by dieticians for 5/2 diet

Whole grains: whole grains are rich in fiber and vitamins,they help you to be full-fledged and content. Carbohydrates is also good food for brain, so whole-wheat bread, durum wheat pasta, brown rice, quinoa and other delicious grains take healthy place in 5/2 ration.

Vegetables: broccoli, cauliflower, Brussels sprouts zucchinis, and other is a fair play on 5/2 diet. Generously load your place with varicolored vegetables to obtain all useful properties.

Fruits: fruits take considerable place in every diet. You can enjoy citruses, berries, apples (avoid bananas-they are too caloric)

High-fiber products: beans, lentil, oatmeal, buckwheat, sprouted grains.

Healthy fats: compulsory add in your ration seeds, olive/sesame/flaxseed oil, avocado, fat fish and other omega 3 and omega 6 sources. It will give your body energy when it has lack of glycogen stocks.

Lean proteins: such products like chicken breast, turkey, eggs, fish, may provide you with steady energy and protein which is essential for your organism for muscle growing and cell regeneration.

Red meat: although it's better stick to lean meat during diets, several pieces of red meat won't be harmful. Try to add non-fat minced beef or low-fat fillet steak.

Beverages: you may drink everything you want in your usual days but it's better to drink non caloric beverages during fasting days. Try to drink a lot of water, sugar-free juices, chamomile tea.

Tips

- It is desirable to take notes of what you have eaten-it is a comfortable way to keep yourself under the control. You can download an app for your smartphone calorie calculator.
- You may eat all fruits except banana and avocado. They are extremely caloric.
- When you feel hunger it is better to have a cup of water and only in half an hour you may eat
- If you grab a bite with nuts or seeds it will help you to stay done for a long time
- Yoga, swimming pool, fitness, Pilates and other physical activity will help to boost up effect.
- You don't have to hit on sausages, chocolate or buns, it's better to intake light salads, soups, vegetables
- You can choose apple, grapefruit or tangerine for a snack.
- It is recommended to eat green pea, spinach, arugula, Brussels sprouts.

Advantages of this diet

- Approximately the whole week you can eat properly, fasting takes for 2 days
- You don't have to starve, you can eat low calorie products based on 500 calories

- You can choose on your own when to cut down the ration it is quite convenient
- Meat, chicken, cheese or bread are not forbidden, you can consume them moderately
- Nerve breakdowns are practically absent
- The risk of diabetes, oncological diseases, and heart strokes is reduced.
- Equal fat loss on account fat not on muscle mass
- Universality and simplicity in keeping this diet which calculated on 2 days
- Fat loss process is not stopped, and takes place gradually at the time of following long-term methodology.
- Absence of a rough control in the ration of your nutrition

Disadvantages

- At the time of fasting you can experience a light weakness
- There is a possibility of accident/random overeating

Contraindications

This diet is not recommended for people having problems with gastrointestinal tract, ulcer and gastritis. Also it is forbidden for breastfeeding mothers, children and teenagers and people who experience inflammation process. If your organs are doing well anyway before sticking to this diet you should consult with a doctor.

Examples of menu for 2 days

Plan 1

1day(490kcal)

Breakfast(190kcal)-1 portion oatmeal on water,40g whole wheat cornflakes, 1 apple

Dinner(300kcal)-chicken grilled or steamed fillet with adding of olive oil and spices,1 orrange.

2 day(500kcal)

Breakfast(290kcal)- omelet(2eggs),30g cheese and 1 tomato

Dinner(210kcal)-100 non-fat steamed fish,1/2 orrange

Plan 2

1 day (500kcal)

Breakfast (200kcal)-2 boiled eggs, 1 rye crust

Dinner (300kcal)-cream broccoli soup with spices and herbs, 100g boiled fillet with vegetables.

2day (550 kcal)

Breakfast (200kcal)-200g non-fat cottage cheese, 1 orange

Dinner (350kcal)-1 bran crust, 1bacon slice,30g cheese,100g boiled rice with 70g seafood and cherry tomatoes.

Plan 3

1 day (460 kcal)
Breakfast (250kcal) 1 boiled egg, 50g non-fat cottage cheese, 1 persimmon
Dinner (210kcal) vegetable cream soup, 100g baked chicken breast, 50g green pea
2 day) 425 kcal)
Breakfast (205kcal) buckwheat porridge, 50g non- fat yogurt, 1 apple
Dinner (220kcal) vegetable soup, 100g boiled non-fat sort of fish, 1 grapefruit

Personal experience

From personal experience Tony Green.

«Being a student I took part in all sport competitions on a regular basis. In my thirties when my career went up and family life took the rest of the time, I couldn't make enough time for physical exercises and monitor what I ate. When I reached 40 I put on more than 16 kg and was completely overweight. During many years I made some attempts to bring back my former shape by doing different physical activity but without significant results.

In March 2013 I watched BBC documentary film by Michael Mosley. It was about diet 5/2 which lies in consuming calories for 2 days per week would be 25% or less than normal daily nutrition.

Comparatively with other diets it seemed much more relevant sticking to this diet during more long-term. 2 days per week I had to eat a little and all other days I could eat normally, it was morally easier to cope with hunger signals realizing that next day you may eat what you long for.

In April I kicked off following 5/2 diet, fasting on Mondays and Thursdays. The first several days were pretty out-of-the-ordinary and weird to the body. I could feel strong starvation signals at meal-windows just as predicted, but in general it was easier than expected to keep this diet without emotional breakdowns.

Firstly I was reluctant to take up exercising during fasting days but in 3 weeks I noticed great result and since then I undoubtedly prefer combine fasting and training because energy stores are better in these days. Within 14 days I observed a great improvement during running. During 1 year I lost 12kg.

Judging from my personal experience I'd like to point out that diet 5/2 gave the opportunity to boost amount of physical exercises and working capacity.

Approximately right away after start suggesting that there happened considerable hormonal-metabolic processes. It can be interpreted as my energetic depots became more accessible, likely, improving hormonal liver reactions and fat fiber.

Also, I made sure that recovery after physical activity was much faster and on the same day I long for running and training again. Actually in the first part of the year I felt myself full of beans and buoyant, and with better overall energy level in fasting days. The sleep improved in fasting period, but sometimes I could wake up and felt hunger sense. Now after 4 years it has become a part of my life and doesn't bother me at all. It budgets my time and money, and I feel myself on 10 years younger. My physical and physical health is much better and I know exactly that my index body mass and fitness have dramatically improved than 4 years ago.

Basically, this experience is supposed to help people who have overweight, diabetes. In particular, if diets are combined with regular physical activity proper nutrition and healthy lifestyle.

«Personally this diet gave me opportunity to boost my physical effort and improve working capacity. Diet plus regular workout have enhanced my overall health condition as it supposed. Now I am on the way to perfect and healthy body and new life with sport and without harmful food, but according to my personal experience I would like to give you some tips when following this diet:

- ✓ If you want to make most of your new schedule, make sure that your meals are of enough size and contain carbohydrates, proteins healthy fats, vegetables and fruits, because food saturates you itself and then you don't need extra snacks.

- ✓ First 2 weeks is the most difficult as soon as you realize that you fast only in two days you will feel more comfortable
- ✓ As you limit your nutrition you should make sure that you receive maximum use of your meals.

So if you fight with extra kilograms or just looking a way to start a trip to healthy and long life, 5/2 diet is an excellent way to lose weight and make you think of what you eat everyday»

GOAL SETTING

Are you ready to lose weight? Of course you have no idea how to start up, bear it and then not to snap.

Goal setting is the very first step in making your personal weight loss plan which helps you to reach desirable effect, improve and sustain your general health condition. Goals help you to focus, to direct you to the next steps and achievements and motivate you because they are an instrument for measuring your success.

Firstly, you should find out what do you really thirst for. To lose weight for good looking, to decrease backache, either to control weight or just to establish healthy food habits and regular workout.

Short-term goals are an integral part of reaching a success. It is when you expect your achievement during several weeks. They are a step to your long-term goal. So if your goal to lose £35 in total, your short-term goal will be to lose £5 in a month. Other short-term goals may vary according to your wishes, lifestyle and schedule. For example

- Buying cookbooks with healthy recipes
- Draw up recipe collection with non-low-fat products from the net

- Attend master class healthy food cooking
- Sport every day
- Use stairs instead of the lift, cycle or go on foot to work or get off the bus a stop earlier and walk the rest of the way
- Healthy habits
- Stop being hesitant and procrastinator. Start to act.
- Get out all harmful food from the fridge and stock up on healthy.
- While buying up make previously shopping list- to avoid extra unintended groceries.
- Read more informative and useful internet sources about proper nutrition.
- Love and respect yourself
- Try to hang loose by taking your mind from hard working lives and change your residence for a while to recharge batteries on fresh air
- Enroll on fitness classes or proper nutritious classes
- Set your idol poster in a room on the wall, it will encourage you to better results and not to give up

Keep in mind that weight loss goals may be also behavior or state of mind goals. These kinds include

- Eat more slowly enjoying every piece of food and realizing that it carries useful properties in your organism.
- Pay more attention to products labels and their list of ingredients.

- Put an end with negative self-conversation, for example speaking to yourself and claiming that you are fat, ugly, you won't succeed or something else. Think positively!
- Change your walking way to avoid food temptations which may be extremely complicated to resist

Behavior change may include something new that you have never experienced before, for example meditation that will help you to decrease stress level and remove bad food habits for comfort. Keep always up with the latest new research regarding diets. And of course concerning weight control and general condition, any physical activity like jogging, walking on foot, cycling is much better than nothing, it will lift your spirit and may give more freedom and lightness in life.

Staying open and broad-minded-means to be flexible-is the pledge of successful changes. It is a matter of time to break old habits and make healthy changes regular. Trying out new things even if they don't include dieting and weight loss will help you to remain open wholly. It can be useful for you to start blogging or magazine about your trip to weight loss, to track down your goals, share results and experience with other people, develop your own nutrition strategy, explore new feelings day to day and look back on your achievements when you need motivation in the coming years.

Be realistic. Don't set yourself for failure. It is supposed to mean to set attainable and down-to-earth goals. For example if you got used to eating convenience and junk food and your aim is to cook healthy dinners every day from scratch ,please make sure that you are able to make time for it, by all means look through your schedule. Don't forget to take into consideration time for cooking, searching recipes and shopping. If now you are not able to make enough time for it, for the first time set your goal not daily but several times per week until your schedule becomes easier or until cooking healthy food becomes daily habit. So following all these recommendations you have all chances to reach your dream and success

Set yourself on healthy food

Proper and healthy food recipes are an essential component of proper diet or healthy lifestyle. There is a great expression «You are what you eat» and confess that not to agree with this statement is hard.

Human body gets almost all essential properties with food and water. The composition of the products and their qualities directly have a great influence on health, physical development, emotional condition, working capacity and lifespan as a whole. It is quite challenging to find similar factor that has similar impact on human organism.

All vital organism functions are related to nutrition. It is the source of developing cells and fibers, their perpetual regeneration, human's energy saturation. Unhealthy diet, both excess and insufficient is capable of doing significant harm to human health at any age. So people should pay particular heed to proper nutrition.

Proper nutrition lies not in sticking to rigid diets and controlling consumed calories, but providing organism with sufficient and nutritious ration that consists of all necessary products meat, vegetables, fruits and wheat. Picking out the ration is one of the most important tasks but equally important is following it daily.

Of course it may seem difficult for the first time to give up all your bad habits straight away. It may lead to a stress and big tension. Occasionally you can allow yourself a piece of cake or chocolate. But most of time you should eat proper food. The best choice is to cook on your own because supermarket food contains a lot of colorings, preservatives and flavorings that wake up your taste buds. Have you noticed that eating for example candies or chips you cannot stop and eat you want more and more? So it will be better to eat a piece of dark chocolate or baked potatoes with vegetables.

So set yourself to prepare every day healthy meal by yourself until it becomes you every day habit.

Aspects to be taken into consideration while dieting

1. **Don't miss breakfast.** Breakfast is the most important meal of the day. It gives you an energy and power on the whole day. The breakfast is compulsory for every person. At the moment of the breakfast the functioning of organism is launched which needs additional fuel for. Most doctors claim that it stimulates working capacity and brain activity. Most people miss breakfast because they follow a diet and afraid of gaining extra weight, which is considered to be a big mistake. Proper breakfast runs metabolic processes that influence on right caloric consumption.

2. **Take lunch along with you at work.** Since now it will be not so easy to find and make time on lunch break. The best decision is to take homemade lunchboxes at work with you.

3. **Dinner is not only scrambled eggs.** There is no need in cooking the same dinner every day on a quick hand. Try to diversify the ration of your nutrition to make it more varied and enriched it with useful properties.

4. **Late-night gorging** . If you start dieting you should forget about it. If something went wrong you can eat an apple.

5. **Home cooked meals-is better and cheaper choice.** As it was mentioned aforesaid it's better to cook by yourself. But when you have a tight schedule you are not able to make time for it. So find some time during the week to make some food in advance and throw in a freezer or refrigerator. The food is ready for some days.

6. **Food while travelling.** If your work involves frequent flights, it's better to take packed lunches. It is a great way to have always food and not to feel hunger sense.

7. **Healthy snacks** and lot of pep in our step. When is working day finally over and you are going in the gym, eat a granola bar, it is packed with mass of vitamins and useful substances. They contain seeds, nuts dried fruits that provide you with energy

30 HEALTHY RECIPES ON INTERMITTENT FASTING + 30 INTERESTING FACTS

1 day

Interesting facts: Have u known that in 100g broccoli are only 35 calories? It is extremely wholesome and is always an integral component of each diet nutrition. It perfectly copes with cellulite. Ballast substances help to remove all slags and harmful compounds out of the bowel. It also decreases cholesterol having tendency to remove androgen fats from the human body. Moreover it is packed with all kinds of vitamins, including beauty vitamin that is responsible for healthy skin and hair condition. In addition it is effective fighting with cancer cells as contains sulfarofosphan that can prevent and protect from cancer. It was confirmed by scientists.

Chicken with broccoli

Preparation time-35 minutes
Servings-3
Kcal-198

Ingredients:

- 3tbsp / 50g soy sauce
- 1tbsp / 20g honey
- 2tbsp / 30ml rice vinegar
- 1.5 tsp. / 24ml sesame oil
- 3tsp. / 25g cornstarch
- ½ cup / 120ml water
- 1lbs / 500gChicken breast
- 2cups / 350g Broccoli
- 2tsp / 30ml olive oil
- 2 chopped garlic cloves
- 2tbsp. / 20g freshly grated ginger

Preparation steps:

1. In a separate bowl mix soy sauce, sesame oil, rice vinegar, honey and half of cornstarch, put aside.
2. Add ½ cup of water in a cooking pot and bring it to boil.
3. Add broccoli and cover with a lid. Boil for 3-4 minutes to softness.
4. When broccoli is being prepared add the rest of corn starch to chicken, salt and pepper.
5. Preheat olive oil over medium heat.

6. Add chicken and fry until crunchy. Add ginger, garlic. Cook for 2 minutes, stirring thoroughly.

7. Add sauce that we prepared firstly and steam for 4 minutes until it gets thick.

8. Serve with broccoli

> **Interesting facts:** tryptophan that is contained in pasta, promotes producing serotonin so-called bliss-hormone, so consuming this product we can lift our mood and get rid of depression. Regular eating of pasta promotes sleep improvement, helps with headaches, struggles with senility and it's signals, stimulates bowel work and cleans up the organism from toxins

Salad with bacon and pasta

Preparation time-35 minutes
Servings-2
Kcal-187

Ingredients:

- ¾ cup / 190g non-fat Greek yogurt
- 2tbsp. / 30g low-fat mayonnaise
- 1tsp. / 15g mustard
- 1tsp. / 15ml lemon juice
- ½ chopped onion
- 2tbsp. / 30g chopped parsley
- 1.5tsp. / 15g garlic powder
- Salt, pepper
- 2 ½ cup 250g / pasta
- 6 slices smoked bacon
- Lettuce
- Cherry tomatoes
- Slices cucumbers
- 1/4cup/ 40g chopped red onion

Preparation steps:

1. Combine yogurt, mayonnaise, mustard and lemon juice to a homogeneous consistency.
2. Add onion, parsley, garlic, onion, salt and pepper. Place in the fridge for 1 hour. Boil spaghetti to al dente condition.

3. Fry bacon until crunchy in a frying pan over medium heat. Place it on a paper towel to remove extra fat.
4. Combine pasta, tomatoes, cucumbers red onion and bacon. Dress the salad with sauce.
5. Season with salt and pepper.

> **Interesting facts:** Have you known that avocado looks like vegetable but is considered to be a fruit. In spite of taste neutrality avocado is delicious and nutritious. It doesn't contain fats that are not metabolized; it has no carbohydrates and can be classified as purely diet product. It contains minimal amount of sugar and no cholesterol. Including these entire benefits avocado is substantial and caloric products so don't hit on it.

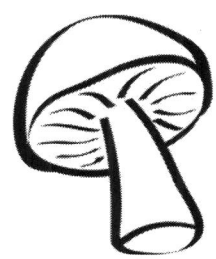

Tuna Avocado Salad

Preparation time-15 minutes
Servings-4
Kcal-363

Ingredients:

- 1 avocado
- 1 ½ cup / 100g Lettuce
- 3 eggs
- 1 can / 600g tined tuna
- 4 Yellow cherry tomatoes
- 2 tbsp. / 30ml olive oil
- 1 tsp. / 10ml lemon juice

Preparation steps:

1. Boil eggs. While eggs are currently being prepared tear apart salad leaves in a bowl.
2. Then get out tuna from the can and dice. (previously remove bones) and add to lettuce.
3. Add sliced avocado and tomatoes the same size. As soon as eggs are prepared, dive into freezing water to make them easily peeled.
4. Cut eggs into 4 parts.
5. Dress salad with olive oil and lemon juice. Add spices to taste.

Interesting fact: Tofu is one of the oldest products on Earth. It appeared in Chine nearly 2000 B.C. Vegetarians and Asian citizens are fond of it. And for good reason, it is nutritious meat substitute and perfect source of protein. . +It is low-fat. It has a lot of iron and calcium and gives more energy to body than meat. It decreases cholesterol level, and likelihood of developing cardiovascular diseases, prevents atherosclerosis and take the edge of cancer risks

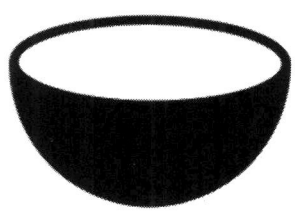

Mongolian Tofu

Preparation time-30 minutes
Servings-3
Kcal-188

Ingredients:

- 3tbsp. / 50g soy sauce
- 2tsp. / 25g natural sweetener
- 2tsp. / 16g cornstarch
- 2tbsp. / 30ml rice vinegar
- 1tbsp. / 7g chopped ginger
- 2 cups / 450g solid tofu
- 2 chopped garlic cloves
- 2tsp. / 30ml olive oil
- ½cup / 30g chopped carrot
- Salt, pepper
- Chopped chives

Preparation steps:

1. Mix soy sauce, sweetener, 1tsp. cornstarch, rice vinegar, ginger.
2. Heat up olive oil in a pan over medium heat. Add the rest of corn starch in tofu.
3. Place tofu in a frying pan and fry for about 4-5 minutes until golden.
4. Add carrot and sauce.
5. Steam for 4 minutes until sauce thickens, stirring from time to time.
6. Scatter with chopped chives.

Interesting fact: Beans are 75% protein, which are close in composition to meat and fish. In beans, there is almost everything that is necessary for normal human health and functioning. That is why beans are considered to be one of 10 the most healthy foods. It is worth knowing that in the process of canning, heat treatment or freezing, all its medicinal qualities are preserved in beans. Only 100g of beans contain about half the daily fiber requirement for an average adult.

Avocado salad with beans and eggs

Preparation time- 10 minutes
Servings-4
Kcal-300

Ingredients:

- 2tsp. / 30ml olive oil
- 1 red bell pepper
- 1 big garlic clove
- 2 large eggs
- 2 cups / 400g dark beans
- 1cup / 200g cherry tomatoes
- 1/4tsp. / 7g cumin seeds
- 1 middle-sized avocado
- 1tbsp. / 7g freshly chopped cilantro
- 1 sliced lemon

Preparation:

1. Heat the olive oil in a frying pan over medium heat. Add red sliced bell pepper and chopped garlic.
2. Break 2 eggs and cover with a lid. Two minutes before preparedness add beans, tomatoes and cilantro seeds.
3. Cover with a lid until substance is heated.
4. Remove the frying pan from the heat and add diced avocado, season with cilantro or any other favorite green vegetable.
5. Squeeze half of lime inside.

Interesting facts Omega-3 fatty acids, which are found in large quantities in salmon, have a positive effect on brain cells, helping to prevent the development of memory and attention problems caused by age or illness. Amino acids help reduce blood pressure, affect cholesterol levels in a positive way, prevent scarring of the walls of arteries and veins, significantly reducing the likelihood of a heart attack. Together with amino acids, vitamins A and D, as well as selenium, fatty acids protect the nervous system from aging, act as natural relaxants, and relax the brain. Salmon is also useful in the treatment and prevention of Alzheimer's and Parkinson's diseases. Perhaps that is why fish lovers are considered more intellectual than meat lovers.

Baked salmon with vegetables

Preparation time- 45minutes
Servings-4
Kcal-180

Ingredients:

- 4 pieces of salmon
- 2 zucchini (green)
- 2 zucchini (yellow)
- 2 tomatoes
- 2onion
- 1 clove garlic
- 1 1/2 tbsp. /24ml lemon juice
- 1 tbsp. /5g thyme (fresh or dried)
- 3/4 tsp. /3g oregano (dried)
- 3 tbsp. /45ml olive oil
- Pepper (ground), salt

Preparation steps:

1. Preheat the oven to 200°C/392°F
2. Prepare 4 pieces of foil. Slice zucchini and onion finely.
3. Place in a separate bowl; add chopped garlic, 1tbsp. oil, salt and pepper. Divide prepared vegetables into 4 parts for 4 salmon slices.
4. Place on prepared foil pieces equally. Put on vegetables salmon pieces, season with lemon, salt pepper, and oil.
5. Slice tomatoes and mix with the rest of onion, salt, oregano and oil 1tsp.

6. Place equally on top of each salmon piece.
7. Wrap up every piece in a foil firmly.
8. Bake 25-30 minutes according to the size of salmon pieces.

> **Interesting facts:** Cheese contains more protein than meat
>
> Protein is an important building material of our body. Each of its cells consists of it; it is a part of all tissues and organs. Cheese contains 20% protein, which is several times more than in meat. In this case, unlike fats, the amount of protein is calculated from the total mass. Proteins must be present in our diet daily. On average, it is recommended to consume protein per 1 g per 1 kg of weight. 100 g of cheese contains an average of 20 g of cheese. Accordingly, it is enough to eat 100 g to saturate the body with the necessary norm and avoid protein deficiency, which is dangerous for the body.

Cheese soup

Preparation time-40minutes
Servings-4
Kcal-185

Ingredients:

- 2 cups / 500ml vegetable/ chicken broth
- 1 cup. / 250ml non-fat milk
- ½ tsp. / 9g salt
- 2 potatoes
- ¼ cup / 10g fresh basil
- ¼ cup / 60g Parmesan cheese
- Ground pepper

Preparation steps:

1. Peel and dice potato.
2. Place it in a saucepan, pour broth, milk and bring it to boil, after add salt.
3. Boil to full readiness of potato.
4. Liquidize soup with food processor.
5. Add basil and cheese. Mix until cheese melts.
6. Season with salt and pepper.

Interesting facts: spinach leaves contain rich in vitamin K.100g fresh spinach contains 42% recommended dosage of consuming this vitamin. It is vital because contributes bones consolidating, stimulating osteotropic activity. Spinach saturates organism with nutrients, removes organism from slags and toxins. It improves metabolism boosts energy. Thanks to high content of iron spinach helps hemoglobin to be more active and provide cells with oxygen better. Regular consuming spinach makes gums and teeth strong and healthy, consolidates blood vessels and normalizes bowel activity and stimulates pancreas work.

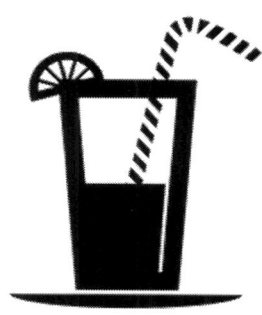

Protein spinach pancakes

Preparation time-10minutes
Servings-16
Kcal-164

Ingredients:

- 2 cups / 450g spinach
- 3 egg whites
- ¼ cup / 30g oatmeal
- ¼ cup/ 65ml almond milk
- 1/4tsp. / 4ml vanilla extract
- 1/5tsp. / 7g cinnamon

Preparation steps:

1. Place all ingredients in a blender till batter condition.
2. If you want you may add a natural sweetener to your taste.
3. Fry on a heated frying pan from each side for about 2-3 minutes.
4. Serve with honey.

Interesting facts: Have you known that pumpkin is a berry, moreover one of the biggest in the world. Its fruits may weigh to several hundred kilograms. Pumpkin is a great product for those who want to lose weight. It is low-calorie, and there are many options for its preparation. Nutritionists advise to include raw and baked pumpkin, as well as pumpkin juice and pumpkin seeds in the diet.

Pumpkin cream soup

Preparation time-30minutes
Servings-5
Kcal-35

Ingredients:

- 1 kg / 3lbs Pumpkin
- 1.5 L / 33oz Water
- 2 onions
- 1 carrot
- 1 garlic clove
- 1 cup / 200 ml cream
- 1tbsp. / 10g butter
- Salt, ground pepper - to taste
- Ground nutmeg - to taste

Preparation steps:

1. Peel pumpkin and carrot, cut into small cubes. Place in a saucepan, pour water and boil to softness.
2. Dice onion and garlic. Fry 1-2 minutes with butter.
3. Combine pumpkin, garlic and onion and blend in a food processor. Add cream to a ready mixture. Stew for some minutes over low heat. Add some water or broth if needed. Add spices to taste. Boil for some minutes.
4. Serve with chopped chives.

Interesting facts: Chicken egg has a high biological value. It contains about 6 grams of protein and all 20 amino acids that are easily absorbed by the body. Egg cholesterol is not dangerous. Eggs have low quantity of saturated fats. They are balanced with useful properties, impending of absorbing cholesterol and contribute to its elimination. Abundant lecithin in egg yolk helps maintain normal cholesterol levels, preventing the development of cardiovascular disease.

Eggs' muffins with black beans

Preparation time- 30minutes
Servings-12
Kcal- 151

Ingredients:

- 1.5 cup / 16 oz. canned black beans
- 1 green pepper
- 1 bell pepper
- ½ cup / 75g red onion
- 8 eggs
- Olive oil
- Salt, pepper

Preparation steps:

1. Preheat the oven to 375F.
2. Place a frying pan on a low heat, add olive oil. Add chopped green pepper.
3. Fry for 7 minutes.
4. In a separate bowl combine eggs, salt, pepper and whisk to a homogeneous consistency.
5. Mix eggs with vegetables, add beans.
6. Divide ready mixture into modes. Bake for 20-25 hours.

Interesting facts: beef is considered to be the most useful and consumed in most diets. Benefits are in a high content of B vitamins, as well as C, E, A, PP, minerals: copper, magnesium, sodium, cobalt, zinc, iron, potassium. Beef is extremely useful for hematopoiesis, is able to increase hemoglobin levels, and is indispensable for anemia.

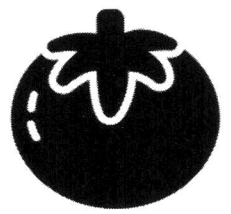

Meatballs with spinach

Preparation time- 45minutes
Servings-15
Kcal- 198

Ingredients:

- 500g / 1lbs non-fat beef/ turkey
- ½ cup / 120g Chopped spinach
- 2 diced onions
- 4garlic cloves
- 1 egg
- 1/2tsp. / 9g salt
- 1/2 tsp. / 8g dried basil
- 1/4tsp. / 4g ground pepper
- 1/4tsp. / 5g oregano

Preparation steps:

1. Preheat the oven to 375.
2. Chop the spinach previously wring out from extra liquid. Chop onion and garlic.
3. Make a mince from meat.
4. Combine all ingredients with hands.
5. Make meatballs and place in a prepared glass mode previously greased with olive oil.
6. Bake for 30 minutes. Cook according to your oven.

Interesting facts: Chicken high benefits lie in easily digestible protein, minimal fat and no carbohydrates. In addition, chicken is rich in phosphorus, potassium, magnesium, iron. Chicken meat can affect blood pressure, participates in lipid metabolism, balancing blood sugar and urine, it also lowers cholesterol and stimulates the kidneys. Chicken meat is an excellent dietary product with low energy value.

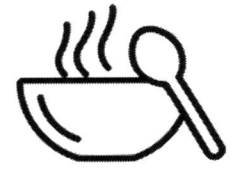

Chicken salad with apples and cranberry

Preparation time- 15minutes
Servings-2
Kcal- 166

Ingredients:

- 4tbsp. / 45ml non-fat yogurt
- 2tsp. / 15g mustard
- 3tbsp. / 45ml lemon juice
- 1/2tsp. / black pepper
- 4oz / 100g boiled chicken breast
- ½ apple
- Celery
- 2tbsp. / dried cranberry
- 1 Shallot

Preparation steps:

1. Combine yogurt, mustard, lemon juice, salt and pepper. The dressing is ready now.
2. Chop the chicken breast, apple and celery. Add sauce. Mix thoroughly to a homogeneous consistency.
3. Leave salad in a fridge for some hours to get more saturated.

Interesting facts: Turkey is packed with a number of vitamins (A , E), as well as in the content of iron, calcium, sodium, phosphorus, potassium, sulfur, iodine, manganese, magnesium. The sodium content in the turkey is two times higher than the beef, so when cooking turkey meat, you cannot use salt. In terms of iron, turkey meat is also a record holder and is far ahead of beef, pork and chicken together. Calcium, which is contained in meat, makes turkey poultry an excellent prophylaxis of osteoporosis, prevents joint diseases.

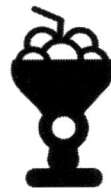

Turkey muffins with broccoli

Preparation time- 35minutes
Servings-12
Kcal- 197

Ingredients:

- 8 eggs
- 1 cup / 175g broccoli
- ¼ cup / 40g chopped onion
- 1 clove garlic, minced
- ¼ cup / 60ml fat free milk
- 300 g / 9oz turkey fillet
- ½ cup / 50g chopped low-fat cheddar cheese
- Salt and pepper to taste

Preparation steps:

1. Preheat the oven to 375. Fry onion until it golden.
2. Add broccoli, garlic, turkey and keep frying over medium heat for 4 minutes.
3. Drain extra liquid. In a separate bowl whisk eggs, milk salt and pepper.
4. Add broccoli, turkey and cheese.
5. Ready mixture divide into modes for baking muffins.
6. Bake 30 minutes.

Interesting facts: A prawn is a low-fat product and extremely rich in Calcium and protein. What's interesting is that the substance that in the process of cooking makes the shrimp red, taking into account all its properties it is 500 times more potent than vitamin E and 10 times and any antioxidants found in vegetables or fruits. Experts have called this substance astaxanthin.

Prawns with rice in tomato sauce

Preparation time- 30minutes
Servings-2
Kcal-210

Ingredients:

- 2 tbsp. / 30ml olive oil
- 2 shredded onions,
- Chives
- 3 tbsp. / 30g flour
- 1 tsp. / 7g garlic (powder)
- 1 cup / 250ml chicken stock
- 1 tbsp. / 7g paprika
- Shrimps
- Salt and pepper to taste
- Rice

Preparation steps:

1. In a non-stick frying pan add flour and olive oil. Stir 6-8 minutes over low heat until brown colour.
2. Add onion, garlic and fry for about 5 minutes.
3. After add stock, paprika and shrimps.
4. Bring to boil, reduce the fire, cover and boil for 10 minutes, stirring from time to time.
5. Serve shrimps with rice.

> **Interesting facts:** Although banana is to considered to be high-caloric product and is not recommended in most diets, rare presence of bananas in your ration will provide you with enough amount of potassium because one banana contains 300g potassium that helps to fight with increased pressure and consolidates heart muscle. In addition bananas 1, 5 times more nutritious than potato.

Banana pudding

Preparation time- 30minutes

Servings-1

Kcal-235

Ingredients:

- 1 banana
- 1.5 tbsp. / 20g chia seeds
- ¾ cup. / 180 ml unsweetened coconut milk
- ⅛ tsp. / 2ml vanilla
- ⅛ tsp. / 2g cinnamon

Preparation steps:

1. Mash a banana with a spoon in equal proportions for 2 cups.
2. Add chia seeds, coconut milk, vanilla and cinnamon to the glass.
3. Shuffle everything until smooth.
4. Leave in the refrigerator for 4 hours. This breakfast can be prepared from the night.
5. Garnish with banana slices and a mint leaf.

Interesting facts: The balanced consuming of vegetables contributes to the normal balance of hormonal levels, the beauty of hair, skin, nails, excellent mood and, most importantly, good health. For those who want to lose weight, vegetables are indispensable, as they are low-calorie foods. They are widely used in cooking, due to their rich taste and ability to combine with other products, thereby contributing to the easy digestion of meals.

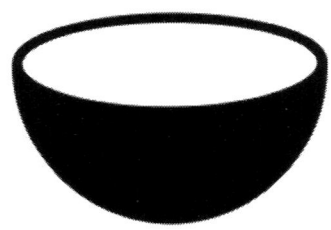

Spaghetti with vegetables

Preparation time- 20 minutes
Servings-3
Kcal-234

Ingredients:

- 3 cups / 300g spaghetti
- 2 onions
- 2 ¼ cup / 400g broccoli
- 3 red bell peppers
- 1 ½ cup / 150g cheese
- Olive oil
- Salt, pepper

Preparation steps:

1. Peel the onion and cut into small pieces. Peel the pepper and scoop out the center with seeds.
2. Cut into small cubes. Heat up the frying pan and fry chopped onion in olive oil until onion gets golden.
3. Add sliced pepper and broccoli, stir thoroughly.
4. Add a little water, salt and pepper.
5. Cook 10 minutes under covered lid, Boil spaghetti to al dente condition.
6. Serve with vegetables and grated cheese.
7. Garnish with chopped parsley.

Interesting facts: Ratatouille a traditional vegetable dish of Provencal cuisine from peppers, eggplant and zucchini. It is also good for an abundance of various vegetables containing many of the vitamins and minerals we need so much, and there are not many calories in it.

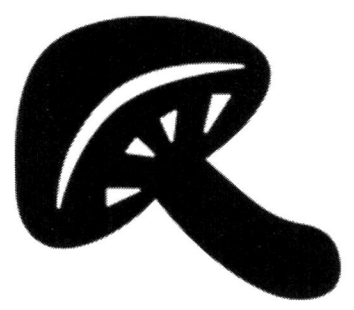

Ratatouille

Preparation time- 30 minutes
Servings-6
Kcal-95

Ingredients:

- 750g / 2 lbs. aubergines/zucchini
- 1 big onion
- 3 celery sticks
- 2 tomatoes
- 1tbsp. / 10g chopped thyme
- 2 tbsp. / 35g capers, drained
- Handful pitted green olives
- 1/2tsp/ 5g tsp. cayenne pepper
- 4tbsp. / 80ml white wine vinegar
- Ground black pepper

Preparation steps:

1. Heat up the olive oil on a non-stick frying pan. It must be boiling hot.
2. Add sliced aubergines and fry for about 13-14 minutes until they get soft.
3. Add a bit of hot water to avoid sticking.
4. Meanwhile place chopped onion and celery with a little of water.
5. Cook for 5 minutes. Add tomatoes, thyme, cayenne pepper and aubergines or zucchini if you don't like aubergines.

6. Cook for 15 minutes, periodically stirring.
7. Add capers, olives and stew for about 2-3 minutes under covered lid.
8. Season with ground black pepper. Garnish with chopped parsley.

> **Interesting facts:** Carrot is very useful: it strengthens nails, teeth and hair, makes eyesight sharp, and skin - smooth and beautiful. There are a lot of antioxidants in carrot that keep the body young and strengthen the immune system.
>
> What is especially interesting, the amount of antioxidants in boiled carrots is 35% more than in raw carrots – they are not destroyed, but multiplied during cooking. Therefore, pastries with this root crop - for example, our carrot cake - is not only tasty, but also very healthy.

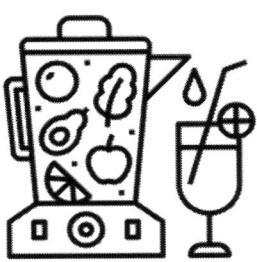

Carrot sugar free cake

Preparation time- 30 minutes
Servings-10-12
Kcal-277

Ingredients:

- 5 ½oz / 150g self-raising flour
- 3 ½oz / 100g ground almond
- 1 ¾ oz / 50g raisins
- 1 3/4oz / 50g walnuts
- ½ cup / 4tbsp. ground mixed spice
- 1 tsp. / 5g bicarbonate of soda
- 3 large eggs
- 100ml / 3½fl oz sunflower oil,
- 3 tbsp. / 45ml low-fat milk
- 300g / 10½oz carrots, coarsely grated

Glazing

- 2/3 cup/ 150g cream cheese
- Zest of 1 orange

Preparation steps:

1. Preheat the oven to 180C/160C Fan/Gas
2. Grease and line the base of a 20cm/8in spring form cake tin with baking parchment.

3. In big bowl mix flour, almond, raisins, walnuts, ground mixed spice and baking soda. Mix thoroughly.

4. In a separate bowl mix all wet ingredients and add to dry stirring to a thick homogeneous batter.

5. Place in a prepared cake tin. Bake for about 35 minutes until it well risen. Insert a toothpick, when pie is ready it comes out dry.

6. Let cool and then take out from the cake tin and top with frosting (stir cream cheese with orange zest) Spread over cake. Cut in small pieces.

> **Interesting facts:** Tomatoes contain a lot of fiber, B vitamins, ascorbic and folic acids, potassium, sodium, phosphorus, magnesium, calcium, iron, iodine, as well as other elements that are important for maintaining health. It is non-fat and approximately 95% of the weight of the tomato is water.

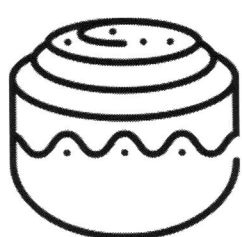

Tomato puree soup

Preparation time- 30minutes
Servings-2
Kcal-35

Ingredients:

- 800g / 2oz canned tomatoes
- 2 garlic cloves
- Olive oil to taste
- Chopped parsley
- 2 big onions
- 1 carrot
- Salt, pepper

Preparation steps:

1. Fry onion on olive oil until it golden.
2. Add carrot and garlic. Fry for more than 3 minutes. Add canned tomatoes. Stew altogether for 7 minutes.
3. Add greenery, season with salt and pepper to taste.
4. Blend with a food processor. If it is too thick add a little more hot water and bring to boil.
5. Serve with sour cream.

Interesting facts: The protein content in lentils reaches 26%, which puts it in third place among vegetables in healthy product list. In addition to protein, lentil is extremely rich in fiber, carbohydrates, minerals and vitamin B1, but almost no fats, calories or cholesterol. The highest fiber content is characterized by green varieties of lentils. Lentils are very useful for women whose iron needs are higher than for men and are recommended during pregnancy.

Lentil with vegetables

Preparation time- 25 minutes
Servings: 4
Kcal-214

Ingredients:

- 1 cup / 200g of red lentils
- 1 onion
- 1 carrot
- 1 sweet pepper
- 2 garlic cloves
- 5-6 mushrooms

Preparation steps:

1. Wash the lentils, pour in water and cook until tender.
2. Lentils boil very quickly. Salt to taste. Fry on olive oil, add chopped onions and carrots.
3. After add sliced red bell pepper and mushrooms. Add squashed garlic frying altogether stirring periodically for 7 minutes.
4. Ready lentil place in a frying pan, stir and cook over medium heat for some minutes.
5. Serve with chopped parsley.

Interesting facts: The best option is to bake food in the oven. In such dishes, almost all useful properties are preserved, and calorie content does not increase due to the large number of oils. When baking, the dish very often emits "juice", in which there are many useful substances. This juice can be poured back into the meat, not forgetting to remove fat from it.

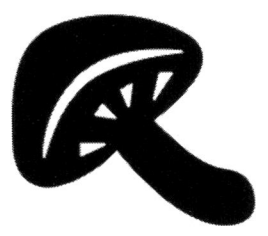

Baked chicken with spinach

Preparation time- 1 hour
Servings: 4
Kcal-224

Ingredients:

- 1lbs / 500g chicken fillet
- 1 onion
- 1 cup / 100g grated cheese
- 2 cups / 250g frozen spinach
- 1 cup /1/3 cup/ 200 ml sour cream
- 3tbsp. / 45ml olive oil
- Salt, pepper to taste

Preparation steps:

1. Cut chicken fillet into 3 parts along. Rub with salt, pepper and spices. (Paprika, ginger.)
2. Heat up the frying pan, fry chopped onion, add squeezed spinach, sour cream, add salt and pepper to taste. Cook over medium heat, until sour cream is thick.
3. Add chopped garlic and a pinch of spicy pepper.
4. Put the chicken in a heat-resistant form, put the spinach on top, sprinkle it with grated cheese and bake for 15 minutes at a temperature according instructions of your oven.
5. Serve with pasta.

Interesting facts: Cottage cheese is one of the richest sources of protein and calcium. It is recommended for those who want to lose weight, as it improves the metabolism of fats in the body, helps in the treatment of heart and liver diseases.

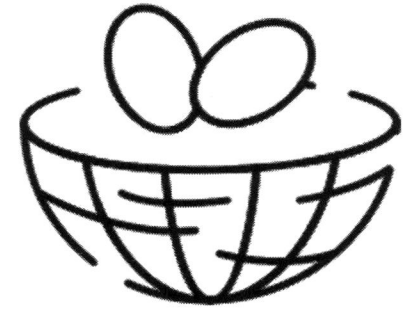

Cheese Casserole with pumpkin

Preparation time- 1 hour
Servings: 5
Kcal-198

Ingredients:

- 2 ¼ cup / 500g cottage cheese
- 2 cups / 300g pumpkin puree
- ¼ cup / 65 ml plain yogurt
- 2 eggs
- ¼ tsp. / 3g cinnamon

Preparation steps:

1. Peel the pumpkin, cut and boil to softness. Then drain the water. Cool down.
2. Place pumpkin in a big bowl and blend.
3. Add yogurt and eggs. Mix thoroughly.
4. Add cottage cheese and cinnamon.
5. Blend again to homogeneous and smooth consistency. Poor in cake tin previously greased with oil.
6. Bake in a preheated to 180°/ 350 F 45-50 hours. Serve with honey.

Interesting facts: It is not recommended eating beans and meat simultaneously, or with fish or dairy products. These products are hard for digesting and beans only worsen the situation. It will be great to combine the use of legumes with fermented products: for example, with sauerkraut (just choose natural sauerkraut - without vinegar and sugar, otherwise it will not be of any use)

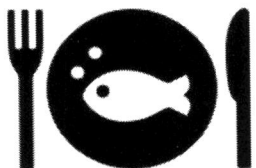

Lean beans cutlets

Preparation time- 35
Servings: 5
Kcal-143

Ingredients:

- 2 cups / 400 g beans
- 1 bulb
- 1 carrots
- 2 potatoes
- salt,
- pepper
- olive oil

Preparation steps:

1. Pour the beans with water and leave for several hours, you can for the night. Then cook until soft, drain from the liquid and cool.
2. Boil carrots and potatoes.
3. Cut onion and fry in olive oil. Pour beans, potatoes and carrots with a blender or grind with a meat grinder.
4. Add fried onion, salt, pepper. Stir until homogeneous.
5. Form the cutlets from the beans and roll them in breadcrumbs. Fry in olive oil on both sides until golden.
6. Ready cutlets can be served in this form, and you can simmer for 5 minutes in a tomato sauce.

Interesting facts: Red pepper contains many vitamins of groups A, C and B, as well as magnesium, potassium and iron. It suits perfectly for people who stick to diets. There are even diets based on this vegetable and help to lose weight. Pepper will help to lose weight due to the presence of fiber and low calorie content. Bell pepper salad can be eaten in the evening without any fear.

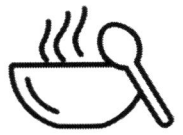

Stuffed peppers

Preparation time- 1 hour
Servings: 3
Kcal-

Ingredients:

- 3 medium sized sweet peppers
- 1 large onion
- 1 chicken fillet
- 2 cups / 250 g fresh mushrooms
- 1 tbsp. / 15ml sour cream
- 1 cup / 100 g of cheese
- Olive oil

Preparation steps:

1. Peel the onion and fry on olive oil until softness. Add chopped chicken breast until it gets golden.
2. Then add chopped mushrooms.
3. Grate cheese. Add 1 tbsp. of sour cream and half of total amount of cheese, mix.
4. Add salt and pepper to taste.
5. Wash pepper, cut in half. Place in a mode for baking.
6. Stuff peppers with ready filling.

7. Bake for 25 minutes in preheated oven to 180. Grate with the rest of cheese and bring back in the oven for 5 minutes more.

8. Garnish with greenery.

9. Serve hot.

> **Useful tip:** To make broccoli soft and tender in a casserole, it needs to be boiled for 5 minutes over medium heat. Previously divide into buds. After drain water and let cool.

Broccoli casserole

Preparation time- 25 minutes
Servings: 6
Kcal-156

Ingredients:

- 2 cups / 300g broccoli
- 4 eggs
- ½ cup / 100ml milk
- Parsley
- 1 cup / 100g Mozzarella cheese
- Olive oil
- Salt
- Pepper

Preparation steps:

1. Whisk eggs with milk until homogeneous consistency.
2. Wash greenery and chop.
3. Place boiled broccoli in a greased heat-resisting mode, sprinkle with greenery and add Mozzarella.
4. Pour with eggs-milk mixture.
5. Bake for 25 minutes in a preheated oven to 180. Grate a bit of parmesan cheese on top. (optional)

Interesting facts: Sandwich is a great way to have a snack. But the most important to choose healthy products to make it nutritious and useful. The main healthy foundation is: whole wheat/rye bread, lettuce, cheese, vegetables and chicken or fish.

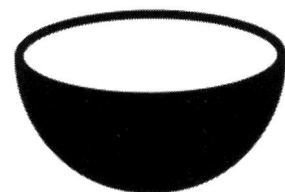

Chicken sandwich

Preparation time- 10 minutes
Servings:
Kcal-118

Ingredients:

- 4oz / 100g boiled chicken breast
- Celery
- Lettuce
- 1/4cup / 65ml non-fat yogurt
- 1/2tbsp. / 7ml lemon juice
- 1 tomato
- Whole bread
- Salt, pepper

Preparation steps:

1. Mix yogurt, lemon juice, salt and pepper. Put aside.
2. Cut celery into small pieces and chop chicken breast.
3. Combine celery and chicken breast with sauce that we prepared.
4. Make a sandwich, on 1 piece of bread put lettuce, tomato slice, and obtained mixture. Leave a sandwich for 1 hour in a fridge and then eat.

Interesting facts: Experts recommend including mushrooms in the diet for people who are overweight, they are considered to be a low-calorie product, quickly saturate the body and satisfy hunger.

Vegetarian rolls

Preparation time- 40 minutes
Servings:
Kcal-112

Ingredients:

- 2 tsp. / 15ml sesame oil
- ½ cup / 75g red onion, ground
- 1 garlic clove, chopped
- 1 cup / 50g of fresh ginger
- 1 carrot, rubbed
- 3 cups / 300g of green cabbage, ground
- 1 cup / 200g of mushrooms sliced
- 1 tbsp. / 10ml soy sauce
- Pita

Preparation steps:

1. Preheat the oven to 300 degrees.
2. Heat sesame oil in a frying pan over medium heat. Add onions and sauté for 3-5 minutes.
3. Add the garlic, ginger and fry for 1 minute.
4. After add cabbage, carrots and mushrooms.
5. Fry for about 3-5 minutes until tender.
6. Add the soy sauce to the pan.
7. Put the mixture evenly into the pita leaves and roll them.

8. Bake for 12-15 minutes until golden brown.

Interesting facts: You may think that there is a mistake, chocolate in a diet? Sounds strange, yes? For sure you have heard different myths about it. «Chocolate causes gaining weight» «Chocolate is harmful», «Chocolate increases diabetes risk» Yes, there is some truth in these words but only when we talk about milk and white chocolate. Dark chocolate is much healthier for human's health. Choose chocolate 80-100%, and where cocoa and chocolate liqueur is on the first place in ingredients' content. A piece (!) of dark chocolate improves brain activity, slows down senility and makes you happier.

Chocolate chip cookies

Time: 30 minutes /
Serving: 16
Kcal 196

Ingredients:

- 1cup / 90g almond flour
- Protein (Vanilla)
- 2 tbsp. / 30g Coconut Flour
- 2 tbsp. / 30g flaxseed flour
- 100 g / 7tbsp. Butter
- 30 g / 2.5tbsp. Erythritol
- 1/2 tsp. / 4g Baking powder
- 1 Egg
- ½ cup/ 100 g Sugar Free Chocolate

Preparation steps:

1. Mix all dry ingredients.
2. Beat room temperature butter with Erythritol until fluffy. Add the egg, beat again. Then add the dry ingredients and mix thoroughly.
3. Cut the chocolate into pieces and mix in the dough. Divide the dough into 16 pieces.
4. Roll the balls, put on a baking sheet and press the bottom of the glass to shape. Send to the oven preheated to 180 ° C/375F for 10-15 minutes, until golden brown. Cool on a baking sheet to room temperature.

Interesting facts: When you have no time to have a lunch, you should predict it because when you stick to diet, organism can't stay without food for a long time. The best choice is granola bar. It contains a lot of cereals and other useful properties that will fill you up and help you to stay buoyant all day long. What should be in the composition of a truly healthy bar? First of all, these are whole grains, dried fruits, vegetables, berries and nuts. These components will provide your body with essential nutrients throughout the day, building materials for the cells and energy to continue your activity.

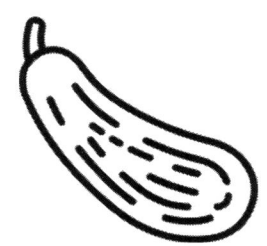

Granola bars

Time: 30 minutes
Serving: 8
Kcal 225

Ingredients:

- 4 cups/ 150g mixture of cereals (oatmeal and buckwheat flakes)
- ½ cup / 50g Peeled seeds (sunflower and pumpkin)
- 1 cup / 150g mixed Nuts
- 7/8 cup / 60g Coconut flakes
- ½ cup / 60g Chocolate chips
- ¼ cup / 35g Nut flower
- 2 tbsp./ 35g butter
- 2 tbsp./ 30g Honey

Preparation steps:

1. In a big separate bowl combine mixture of cereals, coconut flakes and chocolate chips. Add nut flower.
2. Mix butter with honey. Whisk.
3. Pour wet mixture in dry stirring thoroughly.
4. Line oven-tray with parchment paper. Spread obtained mixture by square. It's better to do it with wet hands.
5. Bake for 40 minutes in preheated oven to 160.
6. Get out granola from the oven, let cool completely

Interesting facts: Regular consumption of zucchini in food slows down the process of graying hair and because of their low calorie content; these vegetables are often included in many different diets.

Zucchini casserole

Time: 60 minutes

Serving: 4

Kcal 123

Ingredients:

- 400 g / young zucchini
- 100 g / hard cheese
- 2 eggs
- 100 g / sour cream or cheese
- 0.5 tsp. / baking soda
- 100g / flour
- greenery
- 0.5 tsp. /3g salt

Preparation steps:

1. Grate zucchini, add salt, pepper.
2. Chop the cheese or grate.
3. Mix baking soda with sour cream, leave for 5 minutes, add eggs, whisk.
4. Add flour, cheese and greenery and stir well.
5. Drain extra liquid from grated zucchini.
6. Grease the slow cooker with oil and pour the mixture.
7. Cook in baking mode for 60 minutes.

DISCLAIMER

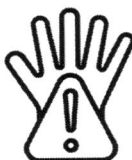

This book contains opinions and ideas of the author and is meant to teach the reader informative and helpful knowledge while due care should be taken by the user in the application of the information provided. The instructions and strategies are possibly not right for every reader and there is no guarantee that they work for everyone. Using this book and implementing the information/recipes therein contained is explicitly your own responsibility and risk. This work with all its contents, does not guarantee correctness, completion, quality or correctness of the provided information. Misinformation or misprints cannot be completely eliminated.

Design: Natalia Design

Picture: unixx.0.gmail.com//shutterstock.com

Printed in Great Britain
by Amazon